10709806

The 48 Laws of contentment

By

Paul A.Reese

Copyright

All rights reserved. No part of this publication may be reproduced, distributed, or transmitted in any form or by any means, including photocopying, recording, or other electronic or mechanical methods, without the prior written permission of the publisher, except in the case of brief quotations embodied in critical reviews and certain other noncommercial uses permitted by copyright law.

Copyright © Paul A.Reese. 2023..

Table of contents

Introduction

We feel contentment, which refers to a state of serene joy or quiet pleasure when our demands are (even briefly) satisfied but we're at peace with ourselves and our surroundings. According to Paul A. Reese, contentment is defined by being "low in activation," having a "strong positive valence," and not worrying. Content people have a great drive to absorb and enjoy.

When we're happy, we often feel comfortable and unpressurized and are working on something personally fulfilling.

For instance, in my idealized version of satisfaction, my cat offers company, my book offers significance and mental stimulation, and my warm, dry home protects me from the chilling rain. After a successful phase, contentment might come when we "stop to smell the flowers" before moving on to other life objectives. Indeed, "mastery activities," or pursuits that foster a feeling of competence, are linked to satisfaction.

Chapter 1

Foundation of Contentment

Being at peace with one's circumstances, body, and mind leads to a mental state known as contentment, which is an emotional situation of satisfaction. Generally speaking, contentment is a softer and more hesitant kind of happiness and may be defined as the condition of having accepted one's circumstances.

A happy person understands that happiness comes from inside, from a pleased mind and a joyful heart.

A person who is happy with who they are and what they have is not searching for or expecting more. The term "contentment" in the moral sciences refers to the absence of greed or excess and insatiable desire. Man tends to satisfy his requirements and suppress his need for more when he has the quality of satisfaction.

In actuality, contentment is a state of peaceful and happy activity. When someone is pleased with their part, they do not feel obligated to exert any effort toward gaining anything.
Being content is being grateful for and content with what you already have rather than focusing on what you desire.

What makes satisfaction so crucial?

It contributes to a calm and developed society, fosters tolerance in the community, and lessens feelings of inferiority among individuals by assisting in the elimination of jealousy and envy in people.

It makes you cheerful all the time and provides you with a calm heart.

Effects of dissatisfaction

THEFT: A youngster who lacks satisfaction would take money from his friends to survive and seem like them. Lack of contentment is a precursor to theft.

PROSTITUTION: Unhappy women are easily seduced into prostitution because they want to buy more jewelry, clothing, shoes, and handbags than they can afford.

JEALOUSY: A jealous individual would seek to destroy the wealthy person to take their fortune. He will start engaging in societal abduction and murder.

Corruption

Greed\Robbery

Chapter 2

Building self-control and wild strength

Good habits are the foundation for success and attaining objectives, and good habits are often founded on discipline, self-control, and the cessation of undesirable habits. But cultivating healthy habits and increasing self-control requires a lot of physical and mental discipline, which is much easier said than done.

Here are five techniques to strengthen self-control and create virtuous habits:

1. Avoid any temptation

According to research, the majority of individuals resist temptation by removing the source of their temptation since we are not equipped to do so consistently.So how can disciplined individuals exist if humans are not born with the ability to control their impulses? They eliminate temptation, making self-control simple. Take action to eliminate the temptation rather than striving to reject it. Manage yourself and your environment by getting rid of temptations to set yourself up for success.

Making choices automated and self-reinforcing enables you to concentrate on matters of primary concern.

2. Monitor Your Development

What is measured is controlled. Monitoring your progress, according to some, helps you stay focused on your objectives. Monitoring makes behaviors easier to control and alter while also assisting us in becoming experts on our behavior.

3.Learn Stress Management Techniques

Your heart rate will drop down if you pause and take a few slow, deep breaths, which will help you unwind right now.

Make sure you receive frequent exercise, a healthy diet, and adequate sleep. Everything enhances your health, attention, and cognitive abilities. When your blood glucose is low and you're sleep deprived, you make bad judgments.

When life and work seem overwhelming, using healthy stress management techniques can guarantee that you have the strength to keep pushing forward.

4. Set priorities

Make a to-do list for each day, week, and month so that you can see your progress and know you're doing your best when you're feeling overwhelmed.

It helps you feel more in control since being disorganized, stressed out, and wasting time are all consequences of feeling overwhelmed and powerless.

5. Pardon Yourself You will fail because failure is a part of everyday life. Moving on requires forgiveness.

It is a waste of energy to criticize and worry yourself; it has no positive results. Success, according to Winston Churchill, "consists of moving from failure to inability without losing enthusiasm."

Your attitude accounts for 80% of goal achievement. A happy worker has a good attitude, so if you want to develop self-control and meet challenging objectives, you'll need to learn how and when to happily grind.

Among the issues that a lack of contentment varieties in our society are the following:

Observe the 48 Laws of Contentment

1. Be pleased.

2. Express satisfaction.

3. Refrain from envy.

4. Avoid jealousy.

5. Be appreciative

6. Embody thanksgiving

7. Aim for independence

8. Stop complaining.

9. Have less faith in other people

10. Take some time to reflect on what makes you happy.

11. Act upon your belief

12. Labor for God, not for your employer or the money.

13. strive towards humility.

14. Pursue the appropriate pursuits.

15 Maintain an optimistic attitude

16. Do not put your hope in people or things.

17. Use healthy comparisons while evaluating others.

18. Change the way you think.

19. Reflect on the promise of paradise!

20. Pray Very Much!

21. Never, not even about the weather, permit oneself to whine.

22. Always see yourself in the current situation; never imagine yourself in any other situation or location.

23. Never judge your situation by another's.

Thank God for the present.

24. Don't ever allow yourself to desire anything else that might have happened.

25. Never think about the future; it belongs to God, not us.

Contentment as a path to happiness

26. Be grateful.

27. Live a life full of love.

28. Discover your mission

30. Stop evaluating yourself in comparison to others.

31. Everyday forgiving exercises

32.Positive companies are also recommended.

34. Never let your inner kid go

Refrain from chasing after worldly possessions.

35. Act with integrity

36. Appreciate the present.

37. Dream big

38. Intention establishes a direction

39. Take enjoyment in little things

40. Accept what is.

41. Exercise and eat healthfully.

42. Zoom out and don't sweat.

43. Laugh, dance, and grin

44. Never stop whining.

45. Never complete a task you've started.

46. Be someone else.

47. Never volunteer to assist someone else because it takes too much time and effort and nobody cares.

They won't be able to express their gratitude to you enough. Nothing is free; life is a marketplace.

48. Always reflect on the past with remorse, rule number

www.ingramcontent.com/pod-product-compliance
Lightning Source LLC
Chambersburg PA
CBHW051728250726
48653CB00008B/3250